THE AT-HOME GYM SERIES

ROWING

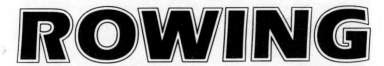

ROWING

THE ROWING MACHINE
EXERCISE PROGRAM
AND
BUYER'S GUIDE

by Michael T. Cannell

Introduction by
Gabe Mirkin, M.D.,
and Mona Shangold, M.D.

VILLARD BOOKS
New York   1985

The instructions and advice in this book are in no way intended as a substitute for medical counseling. We advise anyone to consult with a doctor before beginning this or any other exercise program.

Information on pages 10 and 11 from Helane Royce, *Sportshape* (New York: Priam Books/Arbor House, 1983). Reprinted by permission.

Photographs by Paul Schneck

Produced by The Miller Press

Library of Congress Catalog Number: 84-40601

ISBN: 0-394-72971-4

Manufactured in the United States of America

9 8 7 6 5 4 3 2

First Edition

Thanks to:

Angela Miller
Vincent D'Arrigo
Jean Newhouse
Paul Schneck
Peter Tobeason

CONTENTS

There are numerous basic components to total fitness; among them are strength, cardiovascular fitness, speed, coordination, and muscle flexibility. Any sensible, well-thought-out exercise program will include different types of activities, each of which will help promote the development of one or more of the components of total fitness.

The At-Home Gym Series* presents a wide range of exercises that will help you reach your goal of total fitness. Each book in the series covers a specific activity (rowing, stationary cycling, free-weight training, to name a few), detailing the special exercises and training routines to follow for each. By combining the instructions contained in each book in the series, *you can design your own total-fitness program* . . . you can apply the principles of total fitness and of specific training as you *tailor your exercise program* to your particular goals.

Before you embark on your total-fitness program, it is important to know something of the physiology of exercise.

Exercises can be divided into two categories: *anaerobic exercises*, which focus on improving your muscles, and *aerobic exercises*, which focus on your heart's ability to pump oxygen to the muscles through the bloodstream.

Strength is achieved through short bursts of exercise lasting 30 to 50 seconds and performed against resistance. These are the *anaerobic exercises*, and they include weight lifting, working out on Universal or Nautilus-type weight machines, and sprinting.

The way to make a muscle stronger is to stretch that muscle while it contracts. In weight lifting, your muscles actually stretch before the weight starts to move. The first time that you lift a weight, you use only a few of your muscle fibers. But with each successive lift, you use more fibers until the muscle eventually begins to accumulate breakdown

---

*For other books in this series, see last page of this book.—ED.

products of metabolism and becomes acidic. Since muscle acidity restricts the number of fibers that can contract, you lose the effectiveness of such strengthening exercises after the brief initial burst—10 to 12 repetitions for weight lifters or 100 to 250 yards for sprinters.

Cardiovascular fitness or endurance is achieved through continuous, moderate exercise over periods of no less than 10 minutes. These are the *aerobic exercises*, and they include cycling, rowing, swimming, jogging, dancing, jumping rope, and brisk walking.

In cardiovascular or endurance activities, the heart muscle itself is the one receiving the workout. The body's muscles demand a continuous, elevated supply of oxygen during a workout. Your heart is like a balloon that relaxes to fill with blood and then squeezes this blood from its chambers to the rest of your body. The more blood you have inside your heart when the muscle contracts, the greater the resistance the heart muscle encounters and the stronger it becomes.

Always remember that you must engage in *specific* training activities in order to become proficient in *each area* of fitness. For example, you cannot train for strength at the same time you train for cardiovascular fitness. When you engage in several different forms of specific training, however, you will be well on your way to total fitness.

By acquainting yourself with the basic principles of fitness and by following the guidelines set forth in the various books in The At-Home Gym Series, you can set up and develop your own exercise program without joining a costly health club and without venturing outdoors in brutal summer heat or numbing winter cold. Don't forget to supplement your exercises with the appropriate warm-up and cool-down periods, as outlined in The At-Home Gym Series, and to consult your physician before engaging in any new activity or whenever you are injured.

And enjoy your journey down the path to total fitness!

—GABE MIRKIN, M.D.
MONA SHANGOLD, M.D.

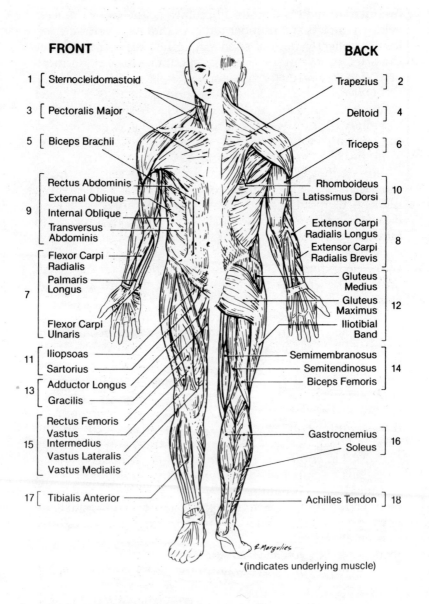

FRONT

1 [Sternocleidomastoid

3 [Pectoralis Major

5 [Biceps Brachii

9 [Rectus Abdominis
External Oblique
Internal Oblique
Transversus
Abdominis

7 [Flexor Carpi
Radialis
Palmaris
Longus

Flexor Carpi
Ulnaris

11 [Iliopsoas
Sartorius

13 [Adductor Longus
Gracilis

15 [Rectus Femoris
Vastus
Intermedius
Vastus Lateralis
Vastus Medialis

17 [Tibialis Anterior

BACK

Trapezius] 2

Deltoid] 4

Triceps] 6

Rhomboideus
Latissimus Dorsi] 10

Extensor Carpi
Radialis Longus
Extensor Carpi
Radialis Brevis] 8

Gluteus
Medius
Gluteus
Maximus] 12
Iliotibial
Band

Semimembranosus
Semitendinosus] 14
Biceps Femoris

Gastrocnemius] 16
Soleus

Achilles Tendon] 18

R. Margulies

*(indicates underlying muscle)

MUSCLE	ACTION
1 Sternocleidomastoid	Tucks chin and rotates head.
2 Trapezius	Lifts shoulders.
3 Pectoralis Major	Pulls arms forward and across the chest.
4 Deltoid	Lifts arms at a right angle to the trunk; assists arms to move forward or backward.
5 Biceps Brachii	Flexes or bends the elbow joint.
6 Triceps	Extends or straightens the forearm and the elbow joint.
7 Flexor Carpi Radialis, Flexor Carpi Ulnaris and Palmaris Longus	Flexes the wrist downward and to both sides.
8 Extensor Carpi Radialis Longus and Brevis	Extends the wrist.
9 External and Internal Oblique, Rectus Abdominis and Transversus Abdominis	Rotates the trunk. Flattens the abdomen.
10 Rhomboideus Latissimus Dorsi	Downward and backward movement of the arms.
11 Iliopsoas, Sartorius	Lifts the thigh and flexes and rotates the hip.
12 Gluteus Medius, Gluteus Maximus	Controls outward leg motion; powers the hip for movement.
Iliotibial Band	Gives lateral stability to the knee.
13 Adductor Longus	Outward leg motion.
Gracilis	Inward leg motion.
14 Semimembranosus, Semitendinosus, Biceps Femoris	Hamstrings; flex the leg and rotate the knee.
15 Rectus Femoris, Vastus Intermedius, Vastus Lateralis, Vastus Medialis	Quadriceps group; extends the knee and flexes the hip.
16 Gastrocnemius	Working together to raise the heel and extend the foot.
Soleus	Constantly in use for standing, walking, running and jumping.
17 Tibialis Anterior	Flexes the foot; changes direction while running and is most responsible for shin splints.
18 Achilles Tendon	Attaches the calf muscles to the heel (the gastroc-soleus group).

ROWING

ROWING YOUR WAY TO HEALTH

The rowing machine, once the exclusive domain of brawny collegiate crewmen, has come of age and is making its way into health clubs and living rooms everywhere.

The rowing machine is the fastest-growing item in the high-tech fitness market boom, and its appeal is easy to understand. Rowing tunes the heart, lungs, and muscles—all with one basic motion. No other sport, with the exception of cross-country skiing, uses more muscles and burns more calories.

Best of all, rowing provides a workout second to none with almost no risk of injury.

Nearly half a million moderately priced rowing machines were sold in the last two years, as thousands defected from running paths and health clubs in favor of the privacy and convenience of exercising at home. As converts are discovering, you can row your way to health in your own living room at a fraction of the cost of joining a health club.

Cardiovascular Capacity

Perhaps the most important aspect of physical conditioning is endurance. Your ability to sustain physical effort for long periods does not depend on the strength of single muscles, as you might think. It's the amount of oxygen supplied to all parts of the body that determines endurance. Working muscles call for oxygen, which can only be satisfied if the lungs, heart, and circulation are in good condition. Your efficiency in delivering oxygenated blood to the muscles is your *cardiovascular capacity.* The heart is a muscle like any other, and grows stronger with training. You'll see measured progress in your cardiovascular capacity as you embark on a rowing program.

Unless you regularly participate in a demanding physical activity, you probably don't know just how much your heart and lungs have slackened off. The next time you go walking, use this test to determine exactly how lazy your cardiovascular system has become. At your normal walking pace, see how many steps you can take on one breath. It's easy to do once, but can you sustain it? Try inhaling for five paces and exhaling for five paces. If you cannot comfortably maintain that breathing rhythm for the duration of your walk, your body has become seriously idle. But it need not stay that way. By improving lung capacity, breathing patterns, and heart strength, you can acquire a resistance to fatigue.

Aerobic Benefit

A rower pulling at peak intensity drains the energy stored in his or her muscle tissue in a little over a minute. Thereafter, energy is metabolized from the oxygen delivered by the blood. Because rowing exercises so many muscle groups, there's a loud call throughout the body for oxygen.

At rest, your heart pumps about five liters of oxygenated blood per minute. A competitive oarsman going at top pace is capable of pumping eight times that amount in order to deliver the six or so liters of oxygen his or her working muscles call for.

This whole process in which your muscles beg for oxygen is *aerobic,* and few sports put it into action as much as rowing. "Rowing is ranked among the highest in aerobic benefit," according to Fritz Hagerman, Ph.D., a physiologist and adviser to the U.S. rowing team. "The energy cost for a given level of rowing is higher than most other sports including cycling and running, because it employs a larger muscle mass. Rowing is definitely among the highest energy-burning activities."

Muscles

Rowing crafts did not always have sliding seats, as they do today. Originally, oarsmen toiled away from a stationary seat. The sliding seat evolved with the recognition that the body is capable of giving out most of its energy through the leg muscles.

The rowing motion, as practiced correctly, puts special demand on the front muscles of the thigh (quadriceps), in addition to the back, shoulder, and arms. It also strengthens the stomach muscles (abdominals) and hamstring muscles at the back of the thigh, as well as the calves and ankles.

When a muscle contracts, hundreds of little strands change form in a process that is at once chemical, electrical, and mechanical. The muscle holds some of these fibers on reserve to be expended later. A muscle develops only when all the strands have been used. If the muscle is stimulated beyond the consumption of all muscle strands, it adapts and becomes stronger. This process is known as *progressive resistance.*

Rowing allows a certain amount of progressive resistance, but it's generally better to acquire strength off the machine than on it. If "bulking up" is a priority for you, you'll want to follow rowing with a weight-lifting regimen. Ten minutes of proper weight training develops more muscle mass than one hour on a rowing machine. A lifting program will, in turn, enhance the aerobic benefit of your rowing program by increasing the oxygen demand on the heart and lungs.

Injuries

Like swimmers, rowers exercise without having to support their body weight. Indeed, rowing is one of the few sports that is good for muscles without putting stress on the joints. That means rowing is free of sore knees, blisters, shinsplints, sprains, and backaches associated with running and other physically jarring sports. Instead of pounding the pavement, your body performs a fluid motion of stretching and reaching. It's ideal for those suffering injuries associated with the jolting punishment of running.

For the same reasons, rowing is a terrific activity for the obese, or people with special orthopedic problems. Exercise is recognized as one of the most potent treatments of arthritis because it pads the joints with muscle. And yet most sports are out of the question for arthritis sufferers. Rowing can help them where running or a racquet sport would be agony. Rowing is beneficial, as well, for the handicapped, or anyone with a neuromuscular disorder that prevents him from carrying weight on his feet.

A clean bill of health is a prerequisite to any fitness regimen. As eager as you may be to get started, it's advisable to wait for the green light from your doctor, particularly if you are older than 35 or have been away from serious exercise for a long period.

Prevent injuries and accidents by being aware of your body's reaction to undue stress and fatigue. Recognize tension and pain as indications that you've exceeded your capacity. That's not to say you've reached an insurmountable boundary on such occasions. On the contrary, by pushing yourself to the limit, and then accepting when to stop, you'll be better equipped to push that boundary the next time around.

Mental Fitness

A chapter on the benefits of rowing would not be complete without some mention of its psychological value. Rowing is, aside from everything else, a chance to unwind. It's therapy.

Fitness, after all, speaks of strength, endurance—and something else: a certain mental attitude of concentration, determination, and inner power. Your mental outlook will brighten as you become addicted to rowing. It's the best possible addiction.

Our everyday duties call not only for physical strength and stamina, but also clear thoughts and mental toughness. Physical and mental health act as partners. It's natural, therefore, that your rowing program should enhance your thoughts and attitudes as well as your body.

There's no *easy* way to make the transformation from a sedentary to an active lifestyle. There are no shortcuts. But the biggest reward, you may find, is how you feel about yourself.

HEAVE-HO! HOW TO ROW

Loosening Up

It's not enough to touch your toes a few times, and then hop straight on the machine. If you take the time to limber up properly before a workout, you'll decrease the chance of injury by improving the flexibility of your joints. The machine itself provides stretching and warm-up, but a rowing workout should be initiated with a range of motions to mobilize and prepare the body.

ARM CIRCLES

Keep the arms straight and swing them from the shoulder in a slow swimming motion. Palms face up as arm goes up in front of you and down as hand passes behind the back. Keep swimming for two minutes.

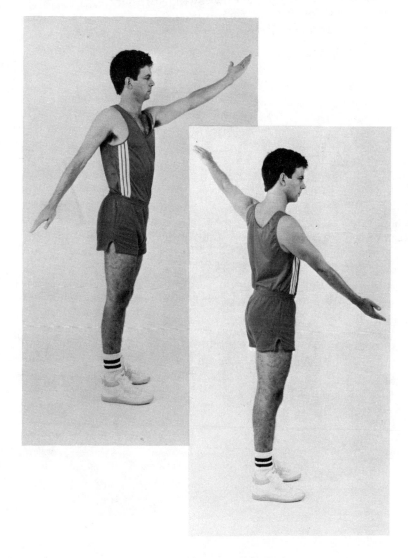

LOOSE ARM SWING

Start with both arms loosely swinging forward and back together, with elbows slightly bent. After two minutes, begin deep knee bends on the downswing. Straighten up on the upswing. Continue for two minutes.

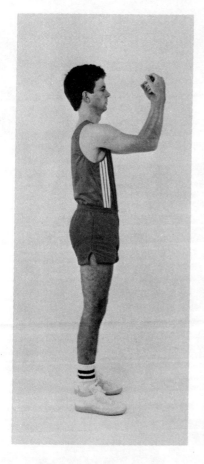
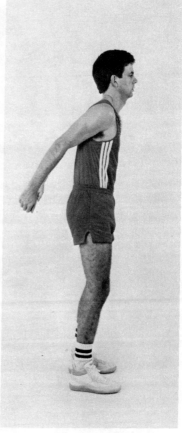

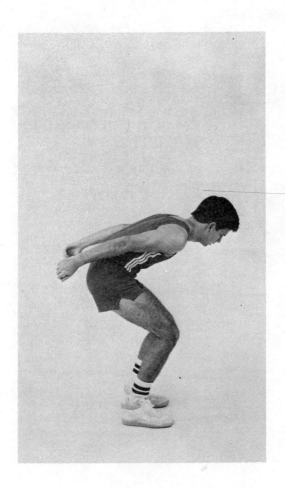

SLOW MARCHING

March in place, slowly bringing knees up to waist height. Continue for two minutes.

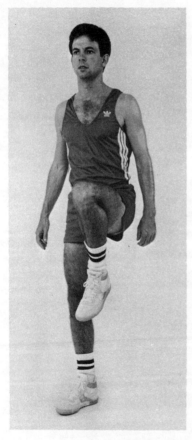 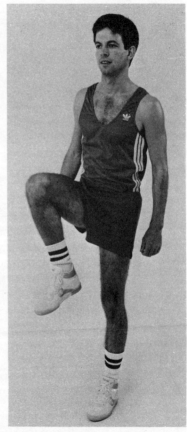

LEG SWING

With one hand on a chair for support, swing leg loosely forward and back from the hip. The motion should be a relaxed kick forward. Swing the leg for two minutes, then switch legs.

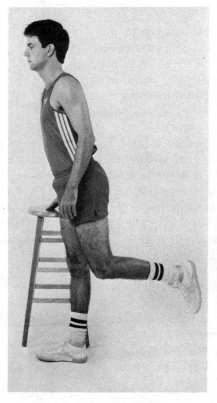
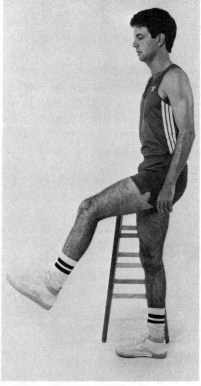

Each exercise should be performed in a slow, relaxed fashion. The goal is to loosen the muscles and joints from your neck to your ankles. These are not stretching exercises, they are simple limbering motions to prepare the body for more vigorous activity.

Go immediately from these loosening exercises to the rowing machine without stopping to rest or do something else in between. If you do stop, you'll lose the limbering benefits of the exercises.

The Rowing Motion

If you're rowing in your own living room, you're not burdened with some of the concerns that preoccupy oarsmen on the water. You don't, for instance, need to worry about "feathering" the oar against the wind, or getting just the right angle in the blade as it drops in the water. And, of course, you don't have to worry about losing your balance and taking an unexpected swim.

As you'll see in the Buyer's Guide at the end of this book, some rowing machines approximate the actual rowing motion more closely than others. But no matter what type of machine you've installed in your home, the principles of the rowing motion are the same.

Skilled instruction in rowing technique is rarely available outside of collegiate boat houses. This guide will show you the basics to help you bridge the gap between your first tentative strokes and a high standard of competence and enjoyment. After all, when you row correctly and efficiently, you'll get a better workout and more enjoyment!

Rowing is more complicated than it looks. The wrong way to row is to sit bolt upright and use only arm motion. The correct way is to use the arms and body together in a smooth fluid motion. Long, slow oar strokes work better than short, quick ones.

The proper rowing motion consists of the following sequential parts: (1) the catch, (2) the drive, and (3) the finish.

The photos show the rower at each of these points. While we can break rowing up into parts and talk about them, the actual motion blends these parts together into one smooth and continuous action. Remember, the word "loose" is probably used by rowing coaches more than any other word. That doesn't mean you should be like a jellyfish. It only means that properly executed, each rowing movement runs imperceptibly into the next.

THE CATCH

The catch is the fully compressed state, beyond which any further movement would be downward, rather than forward. Your legs and body should be in a state of tension, momentarily poised before the backward drive begins. Your knees should be fully bent, with your upper legs just off the chest. Arms are straight and shoulders relaxed.

Make sure the handles are held with the fingers and part of the palm grasped below the knuckles, rather than in the palm alone.

Try to maintain the elbows in an outward position at the same height throughout the stroke. If you let the elbows drop, you'll end up with arched wrists, in the position of a dog begging for a bone.

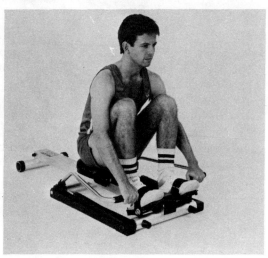

THE DRIVE

The drive is initiated by the legs and back together. As the legs push backward, so does your torso. Both body and leg movements should start together to open up the angle between the thighs and the stomach. Be sure to keep the back straight as you lean back from the hip.

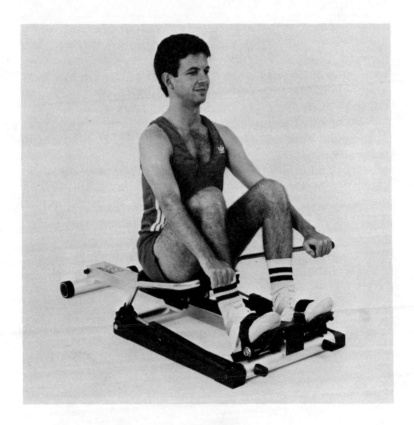

Halfway through the drive, the legs and body are still working together. At this point the arms begin to bring the handle toward the stomach, several inches above the navel. On machines with one handle, aim for this spot early on, because you'll be unable to change direction in mid-stroke.

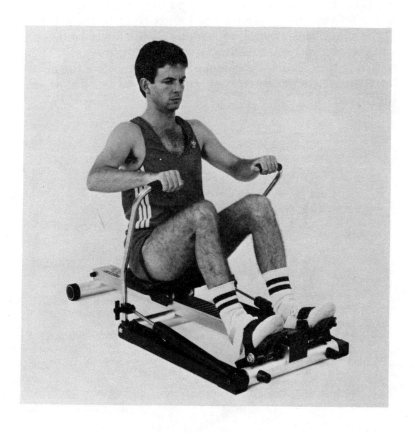

THE FINISH

Bend the arms until the elbows pass on either side of the chest, and the handle is about an inch from the stomach. Make sure the wrists are flat, as they should be throughout the stroke. The sequence of finishing is apt to be legs, body, and then arms, since that is the order of relative strength among these three parts of the body. The arm motion should just start as the legs reach a fully extended position.

After the finish the arms extend forward and the body slides forward as it follows the hands back to the catch. Think of the legs as shock absorbers as the knees come up and you pull yourself back into a coiled-spring position. The return to the catch is a moment of relaxation before the next heave-ho. It should be relaxed, and about twice as slow as the drive.

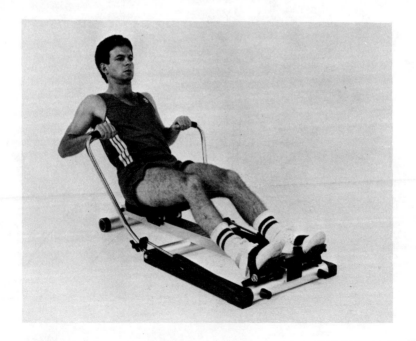

Problems

Even if you follow these instructions closely, you may encounter problems in form and coordination that will hamper your rowing enjoyment and efficiency. Here are some common mistakes:

HUNCHING SHOULDERS

If you have your shoulders up around your head (below), there's something wrong with the position of your wrists or elbows. Sit down at the correct finish position (next page) and row slowly, trying to return each time to a good form at the finish. Be sure to keep your elbows out so your arms can describe a wide motion away from the body. You should support your arms from the upper back around the shoulder blades, not above. Keep the shoulders relaxed.

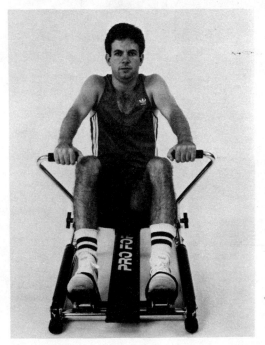

Hunching also occurs as a result of pulling harder with one hand than the other. This tends to happen when you're tired, so concentrate on even strokes at the end of your workout when you're most apt to get sloppy.

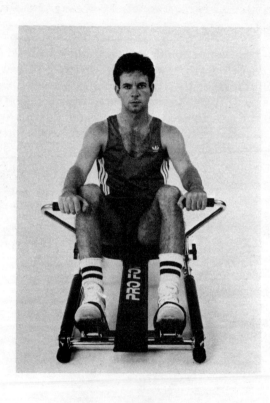

OVERSHOOTING

You're in trouble if the seat stops moving backward before the hands reach the stomach, as in the photo. The farther the handle is from the body when the knees are flat, the more work falls on the upper body alone. The answer is to speed up the upper body action. Don't begin bending your arms until your back reaches the vertical position.

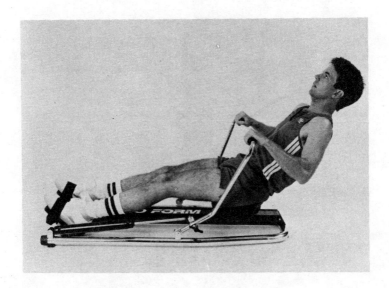

TOO MUCH ARM ACTION

If the arms complete their action before the leg movement is finished, the result will be a jerky motion with too much work falling on the legs. Notice the awkward poise of the oarsman. The legs should be flattening and just finishing their push when the arm motion comes into its own. The remedy for too much arm motion is to speed up the leg action.

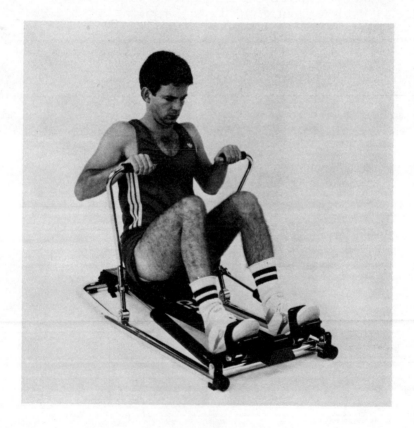

BREATHING

Some people forget to breathe regularly and rhythmically when they get on a machine. Of course, holding your breath makes the work twice as hard. Oxygen is critical to your muscles during exercise. So when you stop breathing, your muscles stop contracting. As you start out, make a point of keeping your head up. Breathe in while gliding forward, and exhale on the drive. Eventually breathing will take care of itself and you won't think about it. But for the first minute or so of each workout, make a conscious point of this "controlled breathing."

Finish with Stretches

The immediate reason for stretching after you row is to discourage soreness the day after rowing. The larger reason is to return the muscles to their normal resting length, thereby improving the joint's flexibility and decreasing chance of injury.

If you don't stretch when you get off the machine, your muscles will develop tightness as they get stronger, and you'll lose flexibility. Eventually you'll develop short, taut muscles, which are susceptible to tears and ruptures. You're better off keeping your muscles at a healthy resting length, and that requires following each workout with careful stretching.

QUADRICEP STRETCH

With one hand on a chair for balance, grab one foot behind you. With your knee pointed toward the floor, not out in front of you, bring the heel in toward the buttocks until you feel the muscle stretch above the knee. This is the quadricep, and it supplies the major power in your backward push on the rowing machine. Hold your foot for one minute, and then switch legs.

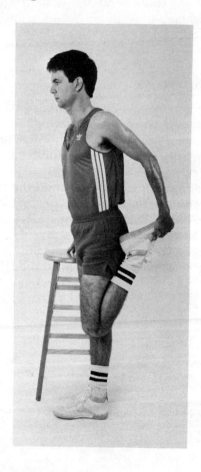

HIP JOINT AND HAMSTRING STRETCH

Lie on your back and clasp your leg behind the knee. Pull your upper leg right into the chest with your knee against the chin. This stretches the muscles across the hip joint. Hold it for a minute.

Next, slowly raise the foot toward the ceiling until you feel the stretch in the hamstrings down the back of your leg. Hold one minute and change legs.

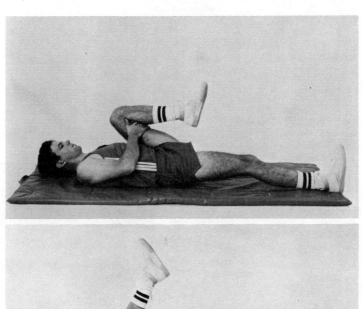

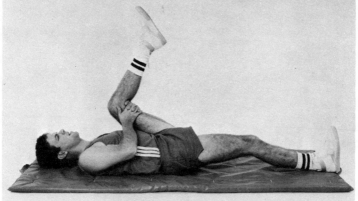

SHOULDER STRETCH

Clasp hands together behind the back, and without arching your back or leaning forward, raise your hands up until you feel the stretch in your deltoids and pectorals and across the top of your shoulder. Hold for one minute.

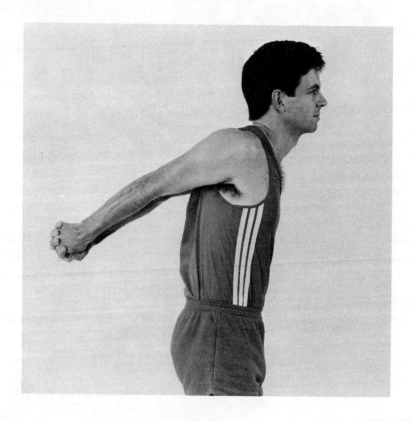

The Rowing Program

Everyone has an internal gauge that indicates the intensity of his physical activity. This gauge is your heart rate. By monitoring your pulse, you can tell if you're exercising as hard as you should be—or too hard.

The goal in your rowing program is to work hard enough to bring your pulse rate up to the zone of aerobic benefit, and then keep it there for the duration of your workout. This is known as **steady-state exercise.**

First, determine your resting heart rate. Press the fingertips of one hand gently to the inner wrist of the other. Can you feel the pulse in the radial artery? Count the number of beats in 10 seconds and multiply that number by six. You now know your resting pulse rate. A man's pulse rate should be 70 to 75 beats per minute, and a woman's should be a few beats higher. If you find your pulse is about 10 beats higher than it should be, it may be due to tobacco or coffee.

Your goal, in each workout, is to work hard enough to raise your resting heart rate to that level which induces the greatest aerobic benefit. That ideal level is your target heart rate, and you want to maintain it throughout your session on the rowing machine.

To determine your target heart rate, first find your maximum heart rate by subtracting your age from 220. This is the danger level of overexertion, and it's a strain on the heart to exercise to this point. Physiologists agree that your target heart rate is 80% of your maximum heart rate. So, if you're 48 years old, your maximum heart rate would be 172. You then multiply that figure by 80 to find your target heart rate at 138.

This is the magic number for you to work toward for optimum fitness benefit. But how do you get there, and how long should you stay? When you get on the machine, you should warm up for several minutes with slow, relaxed strokes. Fifteen to 18 strokes per minute is a sufficient pace for warm-up. It takes roughly five minutes for the cardiovascular system to respond to activity. So increase the intensity of exertion after the initial warm-up, and after five minutes stop to take your pulse.

The heart rate drops quickly when you stop exercising, so be sure to take your pulse immediately, or you won't get an accurate reading. Are you near the target rate? If so, continue rowing at the same intensity for the duration of the workout. If you're above or below it, adjust your exertion level by changing the pace of your strokes, or the resistance level on the machine. Eventually you'll recognize the feeling that is associated with operating at or near the target zone, and at this point you may choose not to take your pulse.

For now, however, monitor your heart rate after the first five minutes of rowing after the warm-up, and once again when you're finished. Be sure to mark your heart rate in your rowing log.

Always cool down before you get off the machine with several minutes of relaxed rowing to ease your heart rate back to its "walking" level. If you step off the machine straight from a full-speed workout, you may experience dizziness or faintness.

Rowing provides aerobic benefit only if you row at least four times a week, and work at or near your target heart rate throughout. Four times a week is the minimum for cardiovascular improvement, but you'll get better results if you can up that to five or six times a week.

For the first three weeks, row for 15 minutes straight without stopping, except to check your pulse. Of course, that 15 minutes should not include warm-up and cool-down at the beginning and end of each session. After five weeks, extend your rowing to 20 minutes. After eight weeks, you should be capable of rowing for 30 minutes without over-straining.

Some machines have various levels of resistance. Find a setting that's comfortable for you, and keep it there.

Rowing machines record workload in various ways: strokes per minute, calories, distance, etc. Learn to work with what your machine has, and keep a record of it in your rowing log. This will allow you to watch your progress and will motivate you toward improvement and new goals.

PULSE RATE

Resting Pulse   Count the beats in 10 seconds and multiply by six.

Maximum Heart Rate Subtract your age from 220.

Target Heart Rate   Multiply your maximum heart rate by .80.

ROWING PROGRAM

1st Workout   Concentrate on technique and motion for 15 minutes. Keep the pace slow, about 15 strokes per minute.

Weeks 1–3   Try to maintain your target heart rate for a full 15-minute workout. You should be operating at 20–25 strokes per minute. Don't forget to record your progress in the log.

5 weeks   You should now have a comfortable combination of pace and resistance to maintain the zone of aerobic benefit. Try a 20-minute workout. If you find yourself straining, lower the resistance level.

8 weeks   Can you go for 30 minutes? Remember: don't skimp on the loosening and stretching exercises!

ROWING
AND
OTHER
ACTIVITIES

Rowing combines aerobic benefit with muscle toning, and thereby provides an outstanding all-around workout. However, if you're interested in developing or strengthening one particular area, you may want to use your rowing program in conjunction with other activities.

In addition, rowing may be used as a training tool to enhance your performance and enjoyment of other sports.

Running

Rowing supplies runners with an upper-body workout that running alone doesn't provide. Also, runners (with the exception of sprinters) tend to have weak quadriceps, which can lead to knee injury. Rowing strengthens quadriceps and can be used by runners to avoid potential knee trouble.

Runners hate nothing more than to miss a workout because of bad weather. Rowing can't improve the weather, but it can allow you to get an aerobic workout without going outside. After all, aerobic training carries over from one sport to another. In addition, rowing calls for the same pacing and mental toughness as running.

Rowing is also an excellent activity for runners who are sidelined with an injury. Rowing is much better for an injured knee or ankle than pounding the pavement, or worse yet, doing nothing at all.

Weight Lifting

As much as it activates major muscle groups, rowing cannot add bulk to your muscles. If muscle enlargement is a priority, follow your rowing regimen with a weight workout. Rowing and lifting can complement each other nicely, since one is aerobic and the other is anaerobic. Together, they develop the cardiovascular system and muscles.

Rowing can prepare the body for weight training by attuning the heart to the workloads to come, and by getting oxygenated blood pumping through the body.

UPPER-BODY EXERCISE

If your goal is specifically upper-body strength, try alternate rowing. This exercise, which can only be done on machines with swing arms, strengthens the biceps, triceps, and shoulders.

Bend the legs slightly and, without moving the seat, push and pull alternately with each arm. For maximum strengthening, perform three sets of 25 strokes.

To develop the biceps muscles, try rowing with an underhand grip, by grasping the handles from below.

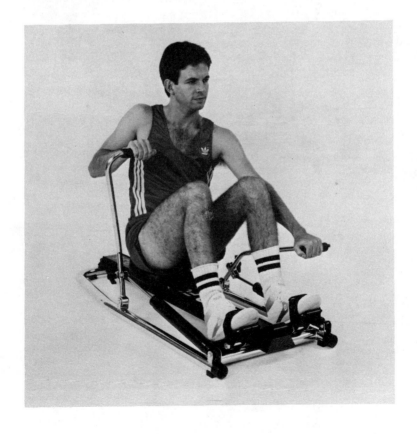

SIT-UPS

If you want to get rid of stomach flab, or strengthen your abdominals, you don't even have to get off the machine. Simply drop the handles, bend your knees slightly, and the rower is a better facility for sit-ups than a "slant board."

Lean back as far as possible, then sit forward and touch elbows to knees. Shoot for 30 repetitions.

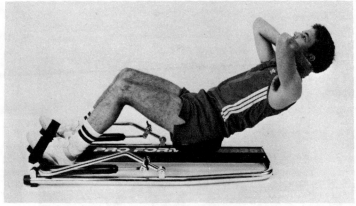

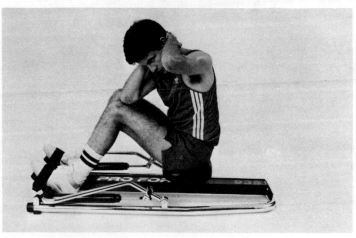

ROWING STRENGTH

Here's a game that tests your rowing strength against another's. Contestants sit facing each other with feet touching and knees up in the catch position. Each person grasps a broomstick and on the word "go" tries to drag the other person forward out of the sitting position.

COORDINATION

Some people seem to have an easier time than others translating a mental understanding of an athletic feat into its corresponding action. Not only does coordination vary from one person to the next, it also varies from one body part to another.

Coordination is not an entirely inborn trait. Muscular skills can be acquired by practice. Rowing is not the most sophisticated of athletic maneuvers, but it can improve general coordination. Rowing sharpens your motor control and this ability spills over to other sports.

BACKPACKING AND HIKING

Most hikers don't have the opportunity to head into the wilderness often enough to keep in top shape. That means when they hit the trail, they're often out of breath and susceptible to aches and injuries. And if they're carrying heavy packs, or moving at high altitude, the problem is compounded.

As an aerobic exercise, rowing is outstanding for improving the "wind." If a hiker prepared for an outing on a rowing machine, it could mean less gasping for breath on the side of the trail.

Rowing also works many of the same muscle groups employed by backpackers. By working the hamstrings and lower back muscles, the rower can help eliminate backpackers' complaints of backaches.

Perhaps most important, rowing keeps the joints in good condition. Therefore, in case of a spill, a slip, or a careless step, there's less apt to be a problem.

TRAINING TIPS

The beauty of rowing is its simplicity and convenience. However, there are a few more things you need to know to enhance your comfort and enjoyment.

Clothing

Avoid tight, clinging exercise attire. A cotton T-shirt and shorts are good for warm weather. For cooler weather, you can try a warm-up suit, or simply add a turtleneck sweater or extra shirt.

Buy yourself a pair of snug, comfortable running shoes. Make sure there's plenty of room for the forefoot and toes.

Keep a towel handy for perspiration. If you find yourself releasing buckets of sweat, you may want to invest in some absorbent wristbands to keep your hands free of slippery perspiration.

Rowing Location

Most rowing machines on the market today are surprisingly quiet. In most cases rowing is inaudible, and won't disturb family or neighbors. However, if you get complaints, try a piece of padding under the machine, or move it to a room with carpeting. Basements and garages are also good locations for you to row without disturbing others, and without others disturbing you.

Depending on the make of your machine, you'll probably have to make some arrangements for storage. Not everyone wants a piece of machinery at the center of his living room. Some machines are designed for easy storage behind a door, or in a closet with the same convenience as an ironing board. Other machines are a bit heavier, and you'll have to learn to live with them in one location. Manufacturers are mindful of this problem, and increasingly are taking pains to style the machines as "fitness furniture."

Music

Music and television are good distractions from the monotony of any repetitive exercise. Some rowers prefer music to television because it enhances concentration. Television has a tendency to absorb all your attention, and you lose track of what your arms and legs are doing. Music with the right beat, on the other hand, can actually help you with your pacing, as well as help the time pass quickly. Choose something fast and upbeat.

Just think, listen to three or four favorite songs on your stereo or Walkman while you're rowing, and your workout is just about over.

Maintenance

Rowing machines have long lives and require little maintenance. Occasionally you may want to wipe it down with soap and water or an all-purpose cleaner. Be sure to avoid abrasive polishes or cleaners.

Check the seat rollers and frame to make sure they're free of dust and dirt. You may want to apply a little light oil to the seat rollers about once a year.

Nuts and bolts should be checked and tightened at least twice a year. If your machine has shock absorbers, lubricate and check the bearings at least once a year.

Important Tips to Keep in Mind

1. Get a clean bill of health before you start the rowing program, especially if you're over 35 or you've been away from exercise for a while.
2. When you stretch, you should feel it. But never strain the muscle to the point of pain.
3. Always warm up and cool down before and after rowing.
4. Don't compare your fitness progress with others. Every individual is different and advances at a different pace.
5. Always work at a heart rate substantially below your maximum heart rate in order to avoid injury and fatigue.
6. Don't hold your breath. Keep your eyes straight ahead and your chin up.
7. Beginners have a tendency to want too much too soon. Don't be discouraged if you can't get into top shape in three weeks.
8. Be aware that tobacco, alcohol, and caffeine will limit the benefits of your rowing program.
9. Enjoy your rowing sessions! After all, it's one thing you're doing just for yourself!

BUYER'S GUIDE TO ROWING MACHINES

If you purchase a rowing machine, you'll largely get what you pay for. Machines are spread over a wide price range, from $200 to over $2,000.

At the top we have the Rolls-Royces of rowing. You'll find these top-line machines, such as the Adams and Gjessing ergometers, only in collegiate boat houses. They're too sophisticated and expensive for home use. For this reason, they won't be discussed in this consumer guide.

Among the remaining rowing machines there are considerable differences in price. How does a buyer account for this disparity when the machines are so similar? Before you make a purchase, carefully consider what you're paying for. Some prices reflect the machine's fancy electronics and sleek "high-tech" look more than good craftsmanship and design.

Still, if you compare the price of the average rowing machine to that of a 10-speed bicycle or a health-club membership, it stands out as a very smart and attractive investment.

This consumer guide is meant to educate you as to what's available. There's no replacement for actually getting on a machine at a sporting-goods store or a health club and trying it out for yourself.

The Concept II Rowing Ergometer
Price: $595
Weight: 49 pounds

This is the favorite of coaches and health clubs everywhere. Its popularity is well deserved. More than any other machine in this price range, the Concept II simulates the actual rowing sensation. The bicycle flywheel works on air resistance, which is similar in nature to water resistance, and approximates the feel of pulling an oar through the water.

It's better for you physiologically, as well, because it calls for a fuller range of motion. You can choose among four resistance settings.

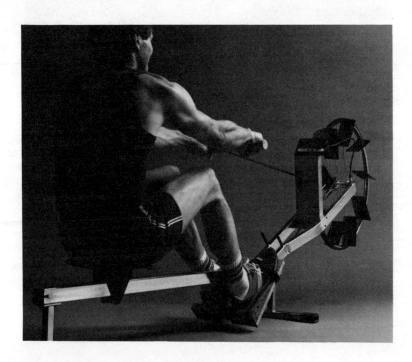

What you gain in authenticity, however, you lose in convenience. It's not a machine that can easily be folded up and put away. But it's narrow enough to be unobtrusive when pushed against the wall when not in use.

An *ergometer* is any machine that records your energy output. A *speedometer/odometer* readout measures your speed and the distance rowed in each workout. This allows you to monitor your performance from one day to the next.

DP Bodytone
Price: $169.99
Weight: 49 pounds

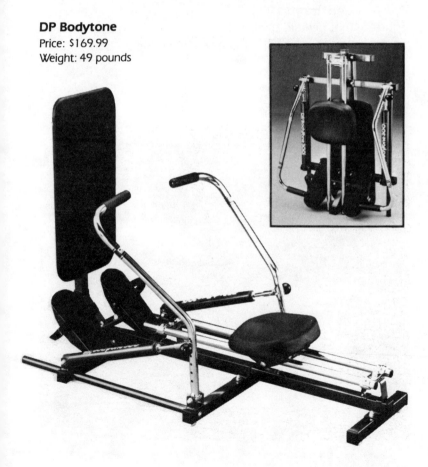

Rowing is only one feature of this multi-purpose device. By folding and turning,this compact unit can also be used for bench pressing, curls, and shoulder pressing. It's light, with a telescopic frame. In its folded position, it can be stored almost anywhere.

The machine's highlight is its adaptability, and not its performance as a rower. It's too flimsy for anyone interested in a serious workout. If you're tall, you won't get a full stroke on this short frame.

A design drawback of the DP Bodytone is the absence of rotating foot pedals. If your heels can't go down as you push backward, you can't get a full or comfortable motion.

AMF Benchmark
Price: $595
Weight: 49 pounds

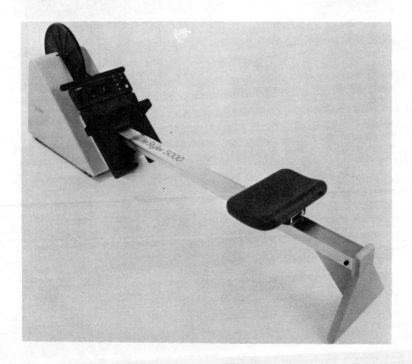

The Benchmark is the latest entry into the rowing-machine market, and not much is known about it. Like the Concept II, upon which it's modeled, this machine has a flywheel that provides lifelike resistance. It has, as well, the same full range of motion and extension on every drive. This machine may be substantially quieter than the Concept II, which is a bit of a clunker.

The Benchmark surpasses its predecessor in the sophistication of its readouts. An electronic system feeds the rower total energy spent in calories, the time worked, and the resistance level. This information is nicely displayed on a digital monitor.

Rowers devoted to the older Concept II will say AMF has made only cosmetic changes—cleaner styling and a modern appearance. However, the jury is still out on this machine.

Precor 630e
Price: $595
Weight: 33 pounds

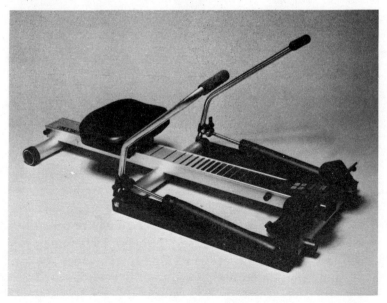

Precor is the most visible and the sleekest of the "swing arm" machines. Unlike the Concept II and Benchmark, the Precor and other swing arms don't require a genuine rowing stroke. Essentially, you're yanking back on a set of handlebars equipped with shock absorbers. The harder you pull, the more resistance you meet. It doesn't require rowing skill, or very much coordination, but still provides an outstanding aerobic workout. If you're more interested in a workout than a rowing sensation, this is a good machine for you.

Welded out of aircraft aluminum, these are solid and durable machines. The design includes a stable, wide base that prevents "leapfrogging" during vigorous workouts. It comes fully assembled with no loose nuts or bolts.

The 630e barrages the rower with more electronic feedback information than a space capsule: elapsed time, stroke rate, total strokes, calories burned per minute, and total caloric expenditure. Most people are able to work out without this information, but you may find it motivates you and helps you set goals.

Precor also produces a similar machine (Precor 612, $295) without any electronic gadgetry, and a much cheaper single-piston rower (Precor 600, $175).

Pro Form 935
Price: $349
Weight: 49 pounds

This rowing machine is similar to the Precor, and is available largely through mail order. It has a durable, heavy-duty base similar to the Precor's, and the same type of pressurized cylinders for resistance. The Pro Form can be stood up vertically to facilitate storage behind a door, or in a closet. Pro Form's drawback is its steel frame, which makes it substantially heavier than Precor.

The Pro Form's electronics feeds you average and maximum speeds, strokes per minute, and miles per hour.

A Pro Form rowing machine is also available without electronics (Pro Form 520, $275).

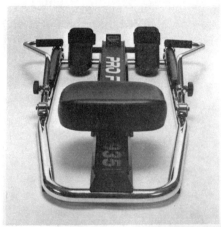

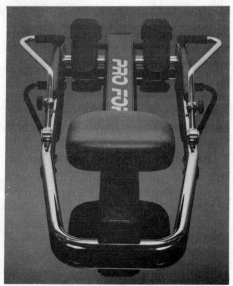

Scandia Hydraulic Rower
Price: $179
Weight: 47 pounds

If you're looking for a no-frills rowing machine, this is it. We see here the same form as the Precor and Pro Form: swing arms and hydraulic pistons for resistance. However, the Scandia is made of a lighter, less durable tubular steel, and the foot pedals don't rotate. The design is hard edged, and not entirely stable.

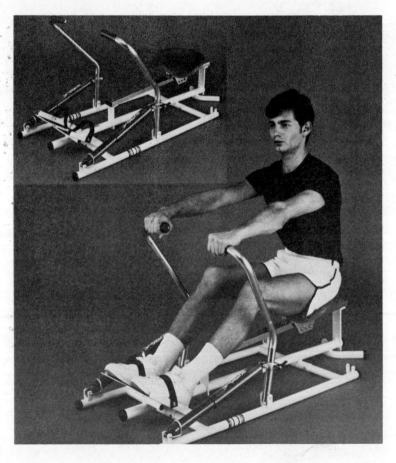

Tunturi Rower
Price: $239
Weight: 40 pounds

The Tunturi was among the first rowing machines designed for home fitness use. While the Tunturi is still a good machine for its price, users complain about outdated design and mechanical problems. It's not a comfortable machine. It's bulky and hard to store.

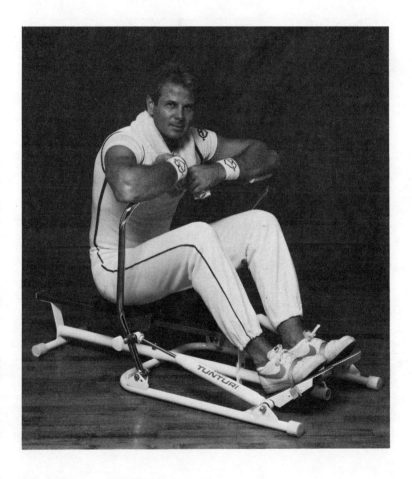

The seat track is thinner than those on competitors, and the seat does not roll smoothly and occasionally sticks. The foot pads come with flimsy straps that allow the feet to come loose and the foot to wobble.

On any machine with handles, your range of motion is determined by the angle of pivot. The Tunturi's design forces you to pull up on the handles, instead of straight back. Some feel that this puts a disproportionate workload on your upper body.

TRAINING JOURNAL

Date	Time	Miles Rowed	Calories	Strokes Per Minute	Heart Rate	Comments

Michael T. Cannell is a freelance writer and competitive sailor who has instructed and coached adults and children at every level. He has been a newspaper reporter, edited two collegiate publications at Princeton University, and has published several articles in *Arts Magazine* and *Streets*.

Mr. Cannell recently completed an instructional book on sailing. He lives in New York City.

VILLARD'S AT-HOME GYM SERIES

( ) 72971-4 ROWING
              by Michael T. Cannell $2.95; in Canada, $4.25

( ) 72972-2 FREE WEIGHTS
              by Judith Zimmer $2.95; in Canada, $4.25

( ) 72973-0 STATIONARY BICYCLES
              by Michael T. Cannell $2.95; in Canada $4.25

( ) 72974-9 WEIGHT MACHINES
              by Judith Zimmer $2.95; in Canada, $4.25

Buy these books at your local bookstore or use this handy coupon for ordering.

Villard Books, Dept. 14-1, 201 East 50th Street, New York, New York 10022

Please send me the books I have checked above.
I am enclosing $ _____.*
For each title, please add 95¢ for postage and handling. Send check or money order—no cash or C.O.D.s, please. Make check payable to Villard Books.

Name_____
                                (please print)

Address _____

City/State _____ Zip _____

Please allow 4-6 weeks for delivery. This offer expires 12/31/85.

*Residents of NY, IL, WI, MD please add sales tax.